Exercise!

It's Now or Never!

Donetta Loya

Author: Donetta Loya
djloya.blogspot.com
Check out her blog for contact information.

Cover: Created with Createspace Cover Creator
Inside: public domain pictures for creation.

ISBN-13: 978-1537092249
ISBN-10: 1537092243

Printed August 2016
In the United States of America

Dedicated to myself!

I deserve to be more physically fit and I need more focus on a healthy body. I feel good, but I want to feel **Great**!

Time for a change!

My health is important.

My physical body balances with my spiritual body.

Find my balance!

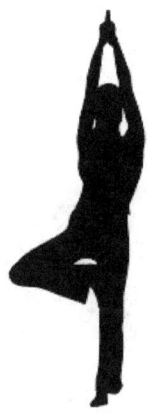

<u>Make the commitment!</u>

I, _____, commit myself to daily exercise and to healthy eating. I will study and plan out a healthier course of action for my good health in the coming year. I will make a real effort each day to make healthier changes.

Signature: _____

Date: _____

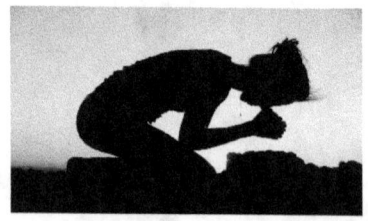

Beginning Measurements:

Hips:_____

Waist:_____

Thigh:_____

Breasts:_____

Arms: _____

Directions:

Weigh yourself at the beginning and then once a week after that. Do not live on the scale. Focus on exercise and eating right. Weight loss is not the only sign of good health.

Date: _____

Beginning weight: _____

Picture of yourself:

(insert picture here)

This is to be a reminder of where you have been....now set a goal of where you want to be!

There is more than just you involved.

There is God...ask him for help.

There is your family...let them know of your goal so they can support you.

You don't have to announce it to the world, but you have to be determined!

It's now or never!

Set your goals.

A goal not written, because a wish.

Set your Monthly goals:

1st month:_____

Goal: _____

Amount of weight loss:_____

2nd month:_____

Goal _____

Amount of weight loss: _____

**Reevaluate goals....food plans, exercise, sleep habits, etc. record them in your weight loss journal.

3rd month:_____

Goal: _____

Amount of weight loss: _____

4th month:_____

Goal: _____

Amount of weight loss:_____

5th month: _____

Goal:_____

Amount of weight loss: _____

Time to reevaluate again. How is your plan working? Time to step up exercise now— don't forget!

6th month:_____

Goal: _____

Amount of weight loss: _____

7th month: _____

Goal:_____

Amount of weight loss: _____

8th month:_____

Goal:_____

Amount of weight loss:_____

How is it going? Are you sticking to your food goals? Find a new exercise routine to break up the staleness....refresh your goals!

9th month: _____

Goal: _____

Amount of weight loss: _____

10th Month: _____

Goal:_____

Amount of weight loss: _____

11th month:_____

Goal:_____

Amount of weight less: _____

*12th month:*_____

Goal :_____

Year mark! How did you do? How much weight have you lost? Time to re-measure your body!

Date: _____

Total weight loss:_____

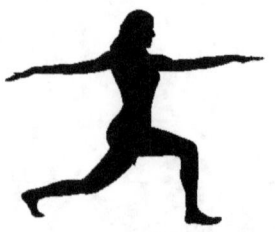

Take new body measurements at the end of your year:

Hips: _____

Waist: _____

Thigh: _____

Breasts: _____

Arms: _____

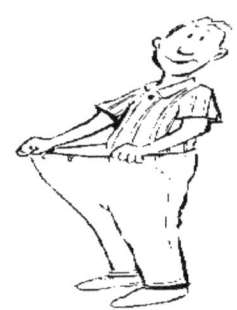

Month: _____

Exercise Chart:

Sun	Mon	Tues	Wed	Thurs	Fri	Sat

Foods: Whole foods **NO Junk foods**!

Lots of water!

Snacking is allowed—If it is a fruit or veggie.

Breakfast: a protein,-eggs lots of ways to cook them!

Lunch: plant food—salad, beans, veggie sandwiches.

Dinner: Little protein, but mostly veggies.

** The other pages have suggestions for meals.

Think smart: Think healthy!

Menu

Evaluate your progress. Write your thoughts, your struggles, your hopes and successes.

───────ༀ───────

*Journaling:*_____

_____

_____

_____

_____

_____

_____

_____

_____

_____

_____

_____

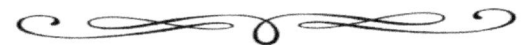

Journaling: _____

_____

_____

_____

_____

_____

_____

_____

_____

_____

_____

_____

_____

_____

_____

_____

_____

_____

_____

_____

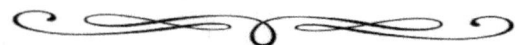

Journaling: _____

_____

_____

_____

_____

_____

_____

_____

_____

_____

_____

_____

_____

_____

_____

_____

_____

_____

_____

Month: _____

Exercise Chart:

Sun	Mon	Tues	Wed	Thurs	Fri	Sat

Foods: whole plant foods *only*!

NO JUNK FOOD. That means no chips, fried foods, candy bars, ice cream...sugared items.

Lots of water!

Snacking is allowed if it is a fruit or veggie.

Breakfast: Eggs—fix in different ways, fruit, oatmeal.

Lunch: Tomato sandwich, Chicken Salad, eggs salad, deviled eggs.

Dinner: Chicken and veggies, Lasagna zucchini, Kitchen soup, Taco salad-no chips.

Evaluate your progress each month. Write your feelings as you exercise daily and strive to eat healthy.

Journaling: _____

_____

_____

_____

_____

_____

_____

_____

_____

_____

_____

_____

_____

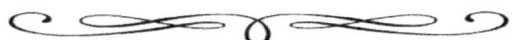

*Journaling:*_____

_____

_____

_____

_____

_____

_____

_____

_____

_____

_____

_____

_____

_____

_____

_____

_____

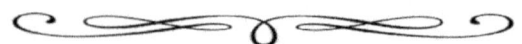

Journaling: _____

_____

_____

_____

_____

_____

_____

_____

_____

_____

_____

_____

_____

_____

_____

_____

_____

_____

Month: _____

Exercise Chart:

Sun	Mon	Tues	Wed	Thurs	Fri	Sat

Foods: whole plant foods

Lots of water!

Snacking is allowed if it is a fruit or veggie.

Breakfast: Tomatoes and toast, poached eggs, Scrambled omelet.

Lunch: tuna salad on wheat bread, ham/cheese roll ups, Salad with boiled egg.

Dinner: Chicken broccoli bake, pork chop, steamed green beans, and ½ potato, meatball soup.

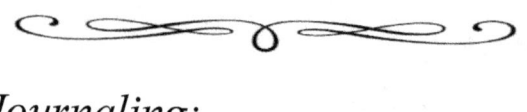

*Journaling:*_____

_____

_____

_____

_____

_____

_____

_____

_____

_____

_____

_____

_____

_____

_____

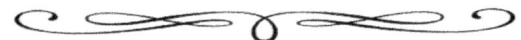

*Journaling:*_____

_____

_____

_____

_____

_____

_____

_____

_____

_____

_____

_____

_____

_____

_____

_____

_____

_____

_____

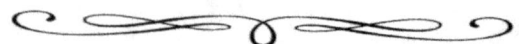

Journaling: _____

_____

_____

_____

_____

_____

_____

_____

_____

_____

_____

_____

_____

_____

_____

_____

_____

Month: _____

Exercise Chart:

Sun	Mon	Tues	Wed	Thurs	Fri	Sat

Foods: whole plant foods

Lots of water!

Snacking is allowed if it is a fruit or veggie.

Breakfast: over easy eggs and hash browns, oatmeal and toast, grapenut flakes and bananas.

Lunch: chicken and sprout soup, salad, fresh veggies dipped in ranch, ham/spinach tortilla roll-up

Dinner: Roast, potatoes and carrots, salad, enchiladas, mini meatloaf and mixed veggies.

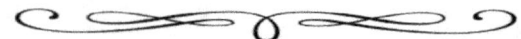

Journaling: _____

_____

_____

_____

_____

_____

_____

_____

_____

_____

_____

_____

_____

_____

_____

_____

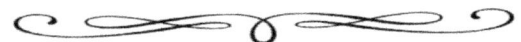

Journaling: _____

_____

_____

_____

_____

_____

_____

_____

_____

_____

_____

_____

_____

_____

_____

_____

_____

_____

_____

_____

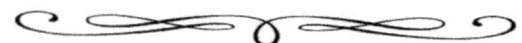

Journaling: _____

_____

_____

_____

_____

_____

_____

_____

_____

_____

_____

_____

_____

_____

_____

_____

_____

_____

Month: _____

Exercise Chart:

Sun	Mon	Tues	Wed	Thurs	Fri	Sat

Foods: whole plant foods

Lots of water!

Snacking is allowed if it is a fruit or veggie.

Breakfast: pancakes with strawberries and yogurt, scrambled eggs and sausage, eggs and toast.

Lunch: tomato sandwich, egg salad sandwich, cheese and pimento.

Dinner: pork chops, mashed potatoes and veggies, tacos and tostadas, chicken ptarmigan with zucchini.

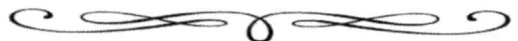

Journaling: _____

_____

_____

_____

_____

_____

_____

_____

_____

_____

_____

_____

_____

_____

_____

_____

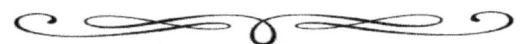

Journaling: _____

_____

_____

_____

_____

_____

_____

_____

_____

_____

_____

_____

_____

_____

_____

_____

_____

_____

_____

_____

_____

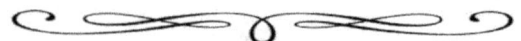

Journaling: _____

_____

_____

_____

_____

_____

_____

_____

_____

_____

_____

_____

_____

_____

_____

_____

_____

_____

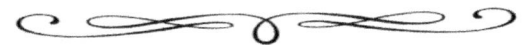

Journaling: _____

_____

_____

_____

_____

_____

_____

_____

_____

_____

_____

_____

_____

_____

_____

_____

_____

_____

_____

Month: _____

Exercise Chart:

Sun	Mon	Tues	Wed	Thurs	Fri	Sat

Foods: whole plant foods

Lots of water!

Snacking is allowed if it is a fruit or veggie.

Breakfast: bird's eyes, eggs and bacon, scrambled eggs and toast

Lunch: grilled cheese and tomato soup, chicken green salad, chopped fresh fruit.

Dinner: Lemon chicken, hamburgers-no white bun, beans and corn bread

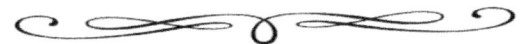

Journaling: _____

_____

_____

_____

_____

_____

_____

_____

_____

_____

_____

_____

_____

_____

_____

_____

_____

_____

_____

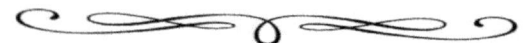

*Journaling:*_____

_____

_____

_____

_____

_____

_____

_____

_____

_____

_____

_____

_____

_____

_____

_____

_____

_____

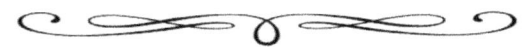

Journaling: _____

_____

_____

_____

_____

_____

_____

_____

_____

_____

_____

_____

_____

_____

_____

_____

_____

_____

_____

Month: _____

Exercise Chart:

Sun	Mon	Tues	Wed	Thurs	Fri	Sat

Foods: whole plant foods

Lots of water!

Snacking is allowed if it is a fruit or veggie.

Breakfast: oatmeal, eggs and toast, eggs and sausage.

Lunch: peanut butter sandwich and jelly, cream cheese and ham tortilla roll-up, chicken salad on crackers.

Dinner: Chicken fajita, bar-b-que chicken and veggies, Bean burritos and fresh pico-de-gallo.

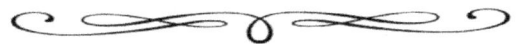

Journaling: _____

_____

_____

_____

_____

_____

_____

_____

_____

_____

_____

_____

_____

_____

_____

_____

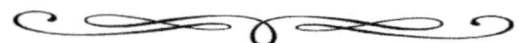

Journaling: _____

_____

_____

_____

_____

_____

_____

_____

_____

_____

_____

_____

_____

_____

_____

_____

_____

_____

_____

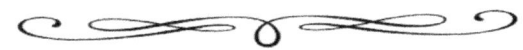

Journaling: _____

_____

_____

_____

_____

_____

_____

_____

_____

_____

_____

_____

_____

_____

_____

_____

_____

Month: _____

Exercise Chart:

Sun	Mon	Tues	Wed	Thurs	Fri	Sat

Foods: whole plant foods

Lots of water!

Snacking is allowed if it is a fruit or veggie.

Breakfast: scrambled omelet with ham, biscuits and gravy and tomatoes, cereal with bananas

Lunch: hot sandwiches with veggies, cheese crisp and salsa, ham sandwich.

Dinner: Stir fry and veggies, Oven fried chicken, red potatoes and green beans, Shepherd's pie.

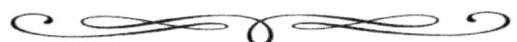

Journaling: _____

_____

_____

_____

_____

_____

_____

_____

_____

_____

_____

_____

_____

_____

_____

_____

_____

_____

_____

_____

_____

_____

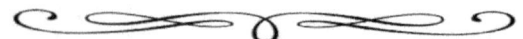

Journaling: _____

_____

_____

_____

_____

_____

_____

_____

_____

_____

_____

_____

_____

_____

_____

_____

_____

_____

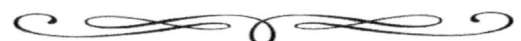

*Journaling:*_____

_____

_____

_____

_____

_____

_____

_____

_____

_____

_____

_____

_____

_____

_____

_____

_____

_____

Month: _____

Exercise Chart:

Sun	Mon	Tues	Wed	Thurs	Fri	Sat

Foods: whole plant foods

Lots of water!

Snacking is allowed if it is a fruit or veggie.

Breakfast: eggs and toast, yogurt and toast, scrambled eggs with bacon bits.

Lunch: Green Salad, beans and cheese, apples and peanut butter dip.

Dinner: Chicken fajita bake, chicken enchiladas, Spaghetti—low noodles and salad.

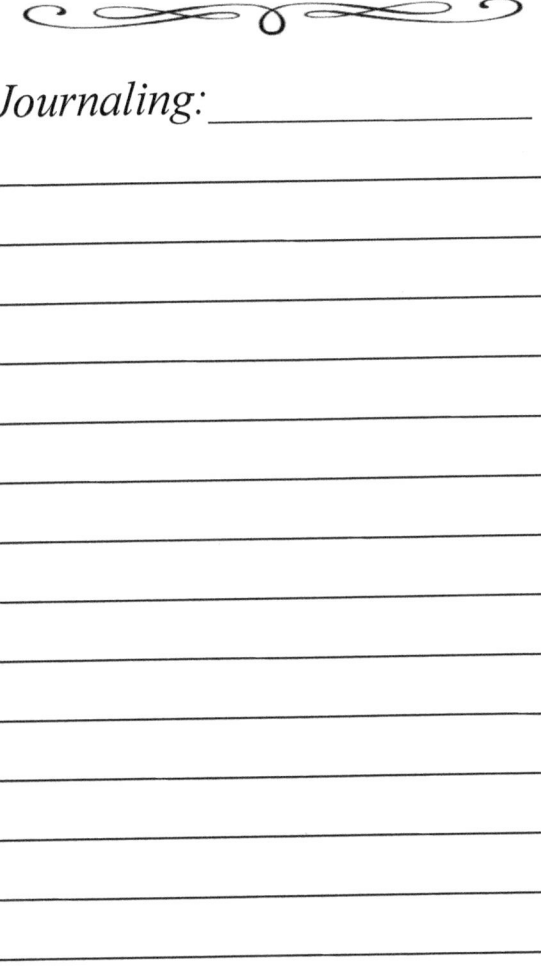

Journaling: _____

_____

_____

_____

_____

_____

_____

_____

_____

_____

_____

_____

_____

_____

_____

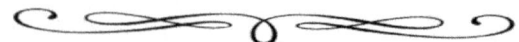

Journaling: _____

_____

_____

_____

_____

_____

_____

_____

_____

_____

_____

_____

_____

_____

_____

_____

_____

_____

_____

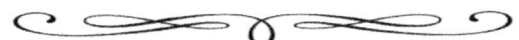

*Journaling:*_____

Month: _____

Exercise Chart:

Sun	Mon	Tues	Wed	Thurs	Fri	Sat

Foods: whole plant foods

Lots of water!

Snacking is allowed if it is a fruit or veggie.

Breakfast: eggs and hash browns, toast and tomatoes, Yogurt and toast

Lunch: Ham sandwich, Cheese and pimento sandwiches, eggs salad and crackers.

Dinner: Beef Stroganoff, spaghetti squash and sauce, stew with veggies

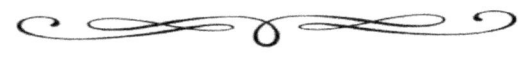

Journaling: _____

_____

_____

_____

_____

_____

_____

_____

_____

_____

_____

_____

_____

_____

_____

_____

_____

_____

_____

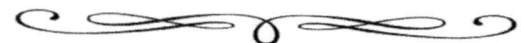

*Journaling:*_____

_____

_____

_____

_____

_____

_____

_____

_____

_____

_____

_____

_____

_____

_____

_____

_____

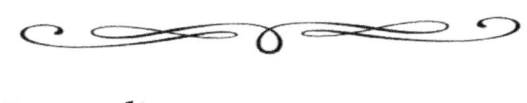

*Journaling:*_____

_____

_____

_____

_____

_____

_____

_____

_____

_____

_____

_____

_____

_____

_____

_____

_____

_____

Month: _____

Exercise Chart:

Sun	Mon	Tues	Wed	Thurs	Fri	Sat

Foods: whole plant foods

Lots of water!

Snacking is allowed if it is a fruit or veggie.

Breakfast: eggs and toast, boiled eggs and fruit, cereal and banana

Lunch: cut up veggies and ranch dressing, Tuna sandwich, ham and spinach roll-up

Dinner: steak and mixed veggies, Baked potato and chili beans with toppings, pork chops and salad

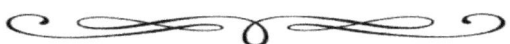

Journaling: _____

_____

_____

_____

_____

_____

_____

_____

_____

_____

_____

_____

_____

_____

_____

_____

_____

_____

_____

_____

Journaling: _____

_____
_____
_____
_____
_____
_____
_____
_____
_____
_____
_____
_____
_____
_____
_____
_____
_____
_____
_____
_____

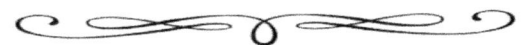

Journaling: _____

_____

_____

_____

_____

_____

_____

_____

_____

_____

_____

_____

_____

_____

_____

_____

_____

_____

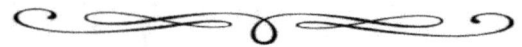

Journaling: _____

_____

_____

_____

_____

_____

_____

_____

_____

_____

_____

_____

_____

_____

_____

_____

_____

_____

Month: _____

Exercise Chart:

Sun	Mon	Tues	Wed	Thurs	Fri	Sat

Foods: whole plant foods

Lots of water!

Snacking is allowed if it is a fruit or veggie.

Breakfast: Scrambled eggs and bacon, fresh fruit and toast, eggs and toast

Lunch: cobb salad, veggie soup, ham sandwich

Dinner: Tacos, roast and mashed potatoes and veggies, fried chicken breasts, red potatoes and veggies.

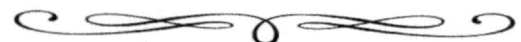

Journaling: _____

_____

_____

_____

_____

_____

_____

_____

_____

_____

_____

_____

_____

_____

_____

_____

_____

_____

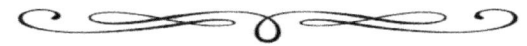

Journaling: _____

_____

_____

_____

_____

_____

_____

_____

_____

_____

_____

_____

_____

_____

_____

_____

_____

_____

_____

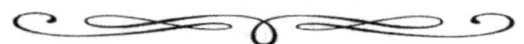

Journaling: _____

_____

_____

_____

_____

_____

_____

_____

_____

_____

_____

_____

_____

_____

_____

_____

_____

_____

_____

Month: _____

Exercise Chart:

Sun	Mon	Tues	Wed	Thurs	Fri	Sat

Foods: whole plant foods

Lots of water!

Snacking is allowed if it is a fruit or veggie.

Breakfast: yogurt and strawberries, eggs and toast, tomatoes and toast

 Lunch: egg salad with crackers, green salad, peanut butter and jelly

Dinner: pizza tortillas, hamburgers, chili beans and cornbread

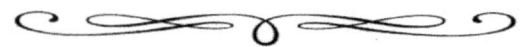

Journaling: _____

_____

_____

_____

_____

_____

_____

_____

_____

_____

_____

_____

_____

_____

_____

_____

_____

_____

*Journaling:*_____

_____

_____

_____

_____

_____

_____

_____

_____

_____

_____

_____

_____

_____

_____

_____

_____

_____

_____

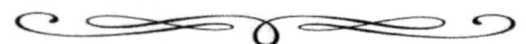

Journaling: _____

_____

_____

_____

_____

_____

_____

_____

_____

_____

_____

_____

_____

_____

_____

_____

_____

_____

Month: _____

Exercise Chart:

Sun	Mon	Tues	Wed	Thurs	Fri	Sat

Foods: whole plant foods

Lots of water!

Snacking is allowed if it is a fruit or veggie.

Breakfast: Scrambled omelet with veggies, fried potatoes and eggs, oatmeal

Lunch: Cheese crisp filled with veggies, chicken stir fry, ham roll-ups

Dinner: Chicken soup, beef stir fry, Taco salad.

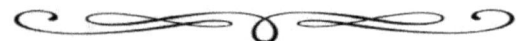

Journaling: _____

_____

_____

_____

_____

_____

_____

_____

_____

_____

_____

_____

_____

_____

_____

_____

_____

_____

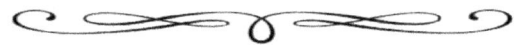

Journaling: _____

_____

_____

_____

_____

_____

_____

_____

_____

_____

_____

_____

_____

_____

_____

_____

_____

_____

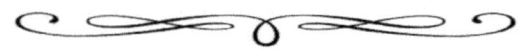

Journaling: _____

_____

_____

_____

_____

_____

_____

_____

_____

_____

_____

_____

_____

_____

_____

_____

_____

_____

_____

_____

Exercise Ideas:

Play your favorite music—soothing, lifting.

First month:

Monday: Beginning yoga stretches

Tuesday: 15 minutes of walking

Wednesday: Yoga

Thursday: 15 minutes of Thigh exercises.

Friday: Yoga

Saturday: 15 minutes of walking.

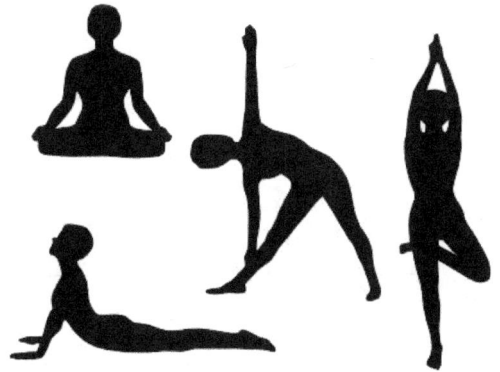

Advance your exercising each month.

Month:

Sun
Mon
Tues
Wed
Thurs
Fri
Sat

Month:

Sun
Mon
Tues
Wed
Thurs
Fri
Sat

Month:

Sun
Mon
Tues
Wed
Thurs
Fri
Sat

Month:

Sun
Mon
Tues
Wed
Thurs
Fri
Sat

Month:

| Sun |
| Mon |
| Tues |
| Wed |
| Thurs |
| Fri |
| Sat |

Month:

| Sun |
| Mon |
| Tues |
| Wed |
| Thurs |
| Fri |
| Sat |

Month:

Sun
Mon
Tues
Wed
Thurs
Fri
Sat

Month:

Sun
Mon
Tues
Wed
Thurs
Fri
Sat

Month:

Sun
Mon
Tues
Wed
Thurs
Fri
Sat

Month:

Sun
Mon
Tues
Wed
Thurs
Fri
Sat

Month:

Sun	
Mon	
Tues	
Wed	
Thurs	
Fri	
Sat	

Month:

Sun	
Mon	
Tues	
Wed	
Thurs	
Fri	
Sat	

Month:

Sun	
Mon	
Tues	
Wed	
Thurs	
Fri	
Sat	

Month:

Sun	
Mon	
Tues	
Wed	
Thurs	
Fri	
Sat	

Thigh Exercises:

First set:

15 sumo squats

10 fire hydrants (Sideways leg lifts)

15 inner thigh lifts (lay down on side and lift knee up to the sky)

Second set:

20 Skater lunges

15 plie squats (ballerina movement)

20 scissors kicks (lay on side and scissor kick your legs.)

Third set:

30 step ups (like on a staircase)

25 side lunges (Stepping to the side and back up.)

30 curtsy squats (like bowing to royalty)

<u>Slimming exercises</u>

On the floor

1. Jack knifes (raise legs up to the sky and over your head) -10 set/ 2 repeats
2. Body crunches (raise knees to your stomach) -10 set/ 3 reps
3. 30 flutter kicks-3 reps
4. Pull knees into chest and extend back out. -15 sets/ 2 reps
5. Sideways Leg lifts (lay on your side and lift the leg on the floor to the roof. -15 sets/2 reps
6. Plank jacks. (put body in plank form, move one leg outward at a time)-10 sets/3 reps
7. Windshield wipers. (lay on back and move your legs out and then in, like opposite windshield wipers.)- 10 sets/ 3 reps
8. Leg lifts- Lay with body tilted toward floor, lift leg up and back, ankle pointed to the sky.) -15 sets /3 reps.

More Exercises!

Standing exercises

1. Leg swings. (Stand up, hold on to a chair, swing legs, in front and then kick back.)- 20 set/ 3 repeat each side.
2. Stand with arms out, bent to touch opposite toe-20 sets/ 3reps
3. Leg lifts. Stand with elbows to chest. Lift legs upward to your chest. 20 sets/4 reps
4. Lunges (take large steps forward, straight back, then stand back up. Repeat each side.) 15 sets/ 3 reps
5. Hold arms out to the side and rotate arms in circles, small to large. Forward then backwards.) 10 sets/ 3 reps
6. Marching (6 steps forward, 6 steps back. Keeping arms raise out to the side.) 8 sets./ 4 reps
7. Wall squats. (lean on the wall while squatting. Hold each one for count of 8. 5 reps
8. Knee lifts. (raise knee to meet opposite elbow and repeat) 15 sets/ 4 reps
9. Walk in place for a full minute. Repeat 4 times.

Exercises tapes are helpful also. Find your favorite to rotate in your exercise schedule.

<u>***Rotate your exercises***</u>—cardio, stretching, muscle building, toning. Don't forget walking! Your body needs the variety. Set up a schedule of your own!

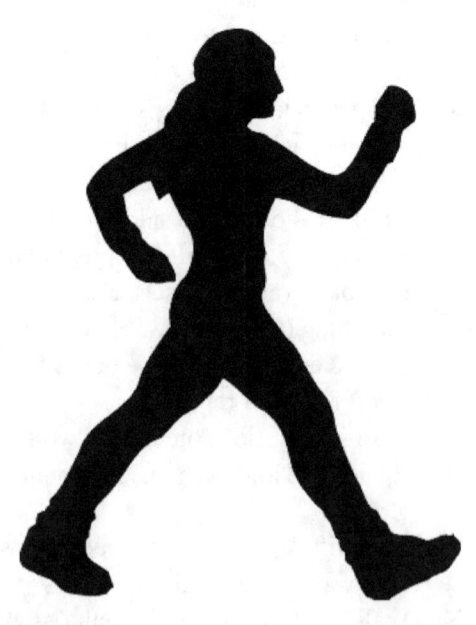

Other activities can give us exercise too. ***Just move!!*** Play sports with the kids. Play tag with the kids! Just keep moving...move more than I did before. All of it is a benefit to my health changes I am making.

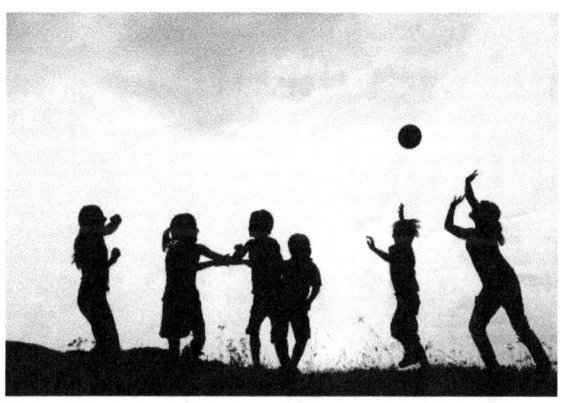

<u>Dance!</u> It is a great way to exercise! Put on music, take a class. Try a new dance video. Dance the weight off!

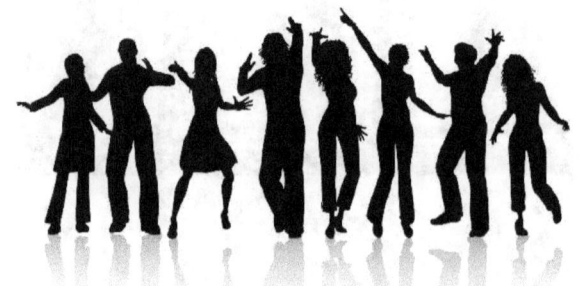

YOGA

Use yoga instructions from Youtube
or get a DVD! Remember books have
informative info also.

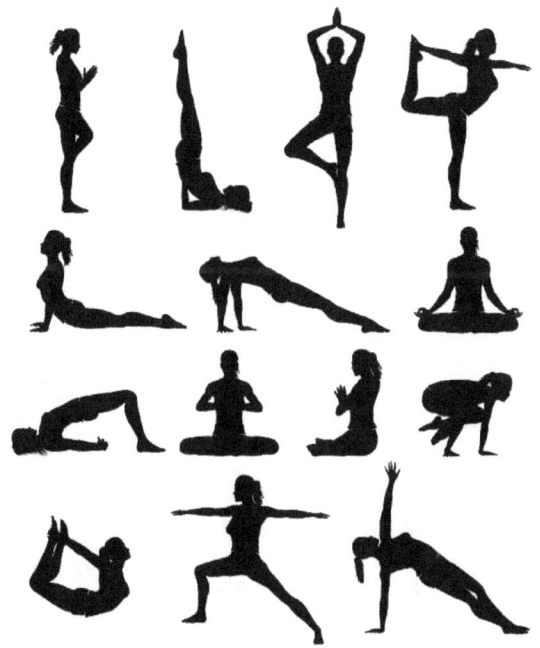

Record Weight, Blood pressure, Blood sugars

Medications:

Record the changes in medication

Notes:

_____
_____
_____
_____
_____
_____
_____
_____
_____
_____
_____
_____
_____
_____
_____
_____
_____
_____
_____
_____
_____
_____
_____
_____
_____
_____
_____